SIMPLE HACK TO CURE ULCER WITH AVOCADO PEAR SEED

CURE ULCER ONCE AND FOR ALL

Prosper Aideyansa Omozuwa

ISBN: 9798324363093

DEDICATION

This book is dedicated to God, for His grace and mercy upon me. Also, to my parents Mr. and Mrs. Francis Daniel Omozuwa, and my siblings, Jennifer Omozuwa, Courage Omozuwa, Merit Omozuwa, and Peculiar Omozuwa.

CONTENTS

ACKNOWLEDGMENTS

First and foremost, my whole gratitude goes to the Lord Jesus for His grace and mercy upon my life then to my family for their unwavering support and encouragement throughout the writing of this book. Their belief in me kept me motivated during the most challenging times. To all those who have contributed, directly or indirectly, to the creation of this book, I offer my heartfelt thanks. Your support has been invaluable, and I am forever grateful.

1

WHAT IS ULCER

An ulcer is an open sore that develops on the inner lining of your stomach or the upper part of your small intestine, the duodenum. The most common type of ulcer is a peptic ulcer.

Peptic ulcer disease

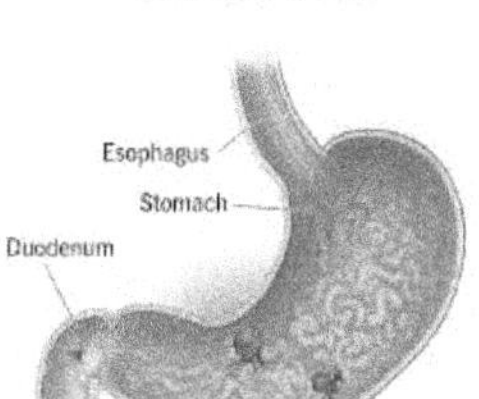

PEPTIC ULCER

Peptic ulcers occur when the stomach acid and digestive juices begin to eat away at the lining of the stomach or duodenum. The lining normally protects itself from these digestive juices, but sometimes the protection weakens and allows an ulcer to form.

There are two main causes of peptic ulcers:

Infection with Helicobacter pylori (H. pylori) bacteria. These bacteria can irritate the lining of your stomach and duodenum, making it more likely that ulcers will form.

Long-term use of nonsteroidal anti-inflammatory drugs (NSAIDs) such as aspirin, ibuprofen, and naproxen. These medications can irritate the stomach lining and increase your risk of ulcers.

Other factors that can increase your risk of ulcers include:

- Smoking

- Drinking too much alcohol

- Caffeinated drinks

- Spicy foods

- Stress

If you think you might have an ulcer, it's important to see your doctor so they can diagnose the cause and recommend treatment. Treatment for ulcers typically involves medication to reduce stomach acid and kill H. pylori bacteria, if present. In some cases, surgery may be necessary, but unfortunately, medication does not completely cure ulcers. That's why this book is written to help those suffering from ulcers for the absolute cure if the instructions are followed carefully.

2

SYMPTOMS OF ULCER

1. Abdominal Pain

The abdominal pain caused by ulcers is often burning, gnawing, or dull in nature and localized to the upper abdomen, just below the breastbone. This pain can range from mild to extremely severe and debilitating. It frequently occurs between meals or in the early morning hours when stomach acid levels are highest. Eating food or taking antacids can temporarily relieve the discomfort by neutralizing stomach acid or providing a protective coating to the ulcer.

However, the relief is often short-lived as the stomach starts producing more acid. The abdominal pain may also radiate to the back or chest, potentially being mistaken for heart-related issues.

2.   Nausea and Vomiting

Ulcers can trigger persistent nausea, especially after meals when the stomach is actively producing digestive acids.

The nausea is often accompanied by an excessive build-up of saliva. In severe cases, nausea leads to vomiting which can induce severe abdominal cramping. Any vomit may appear bloody or have the distinctive coffee-ground appearance of partially digested blood from a bleeding ulcer.

3.   Loss of Appetite and Weight Loss

The abdominal pain, nausea, and vomiting make it very difficult to eat normally. Even the thought of food or the smell of cooking can exacerbate the discomfort.

This lack of appetite frequently results in unintended and potentially significant weight loss over time as the body is deprived of adequate nutrients.

4.   Bloating, Burping, and Indigestion

Ulcers can disrupt the normal digestive process, leading to excessive gas production that causes bloating, belching, and flatulence. There is often a feeling of uncomfortable fullness after consuming just small amounts of food. Changes in Stool

When an ulcer bleeds, even slightly, it causes stools to appear darker in color - ranging from green to black and tarry in texture. In cases of more severe bleeding, there may be streaks or clots of bright red blood visibly present in the stool. This can also manifest as vomiting up material that resembles coffee grounds.

5. Other Potential Symptoms:

- Chronic, dull ache in the back

- Acid reflux and heartburn

- Unexplained anemia due to slow, chronic blood loss

- Fatigue, paleness, and general feeling of illness

While some ulcer symptoms may be mild initially, they tend to become more severe and debilitating over time if not properly treated. Seeking prompt medical evaluation is crucial as bleeding ulcers can rapidly lead to life-threatening complications.

3

THE PRODUCTION STAGE

Processing Avocado pear seed for Ulcer treatment

Below are a few steps to follow in processing the Avocado pear seed:

1. Gather as many pear seeds as you can, at least 10.

2. Wash away the dirt

3. Slice all the avocado pear seed

4. Dry the sliced avocado pear seed under the sun or anywhere

suitable for you After completely dried, grind to powder form

After carrying out the above process for the avocado pear seed, the next step is the application of the powdered avocado pear seed.

The application is very simple, whenever you want to eat, take a teaspoon of Avocado pear seed powder, and add it to your food, do this consistently for 7 days, and that's all.

4

THE DOS AND DON'TS

Dos and **don'ts** while still on this treatment

Dos

1. Begin eating early in the morning, and before you eat take a glass cup full of water.

2. Drink a lot of water (women drink 4 to 7 cups of water a day and men 6 to 11 cups).

3. Eat good food.

4.

Below are some foods that facilitate ulcer pain healing:

- Fruits: Bananas, apples, melons, and pears are good options as they are low in acid and high in compounds that can help reduce inflammation.

- Vegetables: Green leafy vegetables like spinach and broccoli, as well as carrots, green beans, and potatoes are all easy on the stomach.

- Whole grains: Oats, brown rice, and whole wheat bread/pasta provide fiber which can help soothe the digestive tract.

- Lean proteins: Lean cuts of chicken, turkey, or fish are typically well-tolerated as long as they aren't fried or excessively spiced.

- Yogurt: The probiotics in yogurt can help restore healthy gut bacteria balance.

- Honey: Honey has antibacterial properties and can help coat and soothe the stomach lining.

- Green tea: The antioxidants in green tea may help reduce inflammation. Ginger:

- Ginger has anti-inflammatory effects and can help reduce nausea.

- Healthy fats: Avocados, olive oil, nuts, and seeds provide anti-inflammatory fats.

- Probiotic foods: Fermented foods like kefir, sauerkraut, and miso provide beneficial probiotics.

Don'ts

1. No drinking of alcohol

2. No starving

3. No junk food

4. Quit smoking

Below are some foods to avoid while still on treatment, they stimulate ulcer pain:

- Spicy foods: Foods with hot spices like chili peppers, cayenne, and hot sauces can further irritate the lining of the stomach and esophagus.

- Acidic foods: Highly acidic foods like citrus fruits (oranges, grapefruits, lemons), tomatoes, and vinegar-containing items can increase stomach acid production.

- Fatty or fried foods: Foods high in fat like fried meats, French fries, and fast food can delay stomach emptying and increase stomach acid.

- Alcohol: Alcohol can erode the stomach lining over time and increase acid production.

- Caffeine: Beverages containing caffeine such as coffee, tea, and soft drinks can boost acid secretion.

- Dairy products: For some, milk and other dairy items may temporarily relieve symptoms but can also stimulate more acid production.

- Chocolate: Chocolate appears to increase acid production for many people with ulcers.

- Peppermint: Peppermint can relax the esophageal sphincter muscle, allowing acid to reflux up from the stomach.

- Acidic juices: Citrus juices like orange, grapefruit, and tomato juice are highly acidic.

- Processed meats: Items like bacon, sausage, and deli meats are high in fat and salt which can aggravate ulcers.

- Carbonated beverages: The carbonation in sodas and sparkling water can increase stomach acid production and contribute to bloating and discomfort in ulcer patients.

- Certain medications: Some medications, such as nonsteroidal anti-inflammatory drugs (NSAIDs) like aspirin and ibuprofen, can worsen ulcer symptoms and should be avoided if possible.

Following the above instructions is a good way to get to good health.

5

CONCLUSION

The seeds of avocados, which are often discarded as waste, hold promising medicinal properties for treating ulcers. Recent research has revealed that avocado seeds are a rich source of antioxidants, anti-inflammatory agents, and antimicrobial compounds. When ground into a fine powder, this avocado seed powder demonstrates the ability to inhibit the growth of Helicobacter pylori - the bacteria responsible for most stomach ulcers. The powder appears to work by multiple mechanisms. Its antioxidants help neutralize the damaging free radicals that can erode the stomach lining. The anti-inflammatory properties reduce inflammation and swelling around the ulcer site. And most importantly, the antimicrobial effects directly target and kill off the H. pylori infection itself. With its ability to counter the root causes of ulcers on multiple fronts, avocado seed powder may represent a new frontier in affordable, accessible ulcer remedies derived from a highly sustainable plant source. What was once considered an unwanted byproduct could provide relief to the millions worldwide who suffer from this chronic, painful condition.

ABOUT THE AUTHOR

Prosper Aideyansa Omozuwa is one with the experience of ulcer treatment with avocado pear seed, with testimonies from individuals who have benefitted from this simple treatment. The purpose of writing this book is to help those out there suffering from this same issue.

This book is unique because the treatments, by the grace of God, have been tested and trusted by several individuals.